ENLARGE IT!

The Bulletproof Program to Enlarge Your Best

Friend in 71 Hours

Lil Rey

Legal & Disclaimer

The information contained in this book and its contents is not designed to replace or take the place of any form of medical or professional advice; and is not meant to replace the need for independent medical, financial, legal or other professional advice or services, as may be required. The content and information in this book has been provided for educational and entertainment purposes only.

The content and information contained in this book has been compiled from sources deemed reliable, and it is accurate to the best of the Author's knowledge, information and belief. However, the Author cannot guarantee its accuracy and validity and cannot be held liable for any errors and/or omissions. Further, changes are periodically made to this book as and when needed. Where appropriate and/or necessary, you must consult a professional (including but not limited to your doctor, attorney, financial advisor or such other professional advisor) before using any of the suggested remedies, techniques, or information in this book.

Upon using the contents and information contained in this book, you agree to hold harmless the Author from and against any damages, costs, and expenses, including any legal fees potentially resulting from the application of any of the information provided by this book. This disclaimer applies to any loss, damages or injury caused by the use and application, whether directly or indirectly, of any advice or information presented, whether for breach of contract, tort, negligence, personal injury, criminal intent, or under any other cause of action.

You agree to accept all risks of using the information presented inside this book.

You agree that by continuing to read this book, where appropriate and/or necessary, you shall consult a professional (including but not limited to your doctor, attorney, or financial advisor or such other advisor as needed) before using any of the suggested remedies, techniques, or information in this book.

Table of Contents

Introduction to the book

According to research (and perhaps to most women), men often harbor lots of secrets especially when it comes to sex. While they readily admit to these things, they are also quick to point out that most of these supposed secrets that people assume are quite frustrating. One of these "myths" that are going the rounds is that men think about sex 24/7. In defense of the men out there, they often argue that, while their minds do often stray to sex, it doesn't mean that that's all they ever think about. Women, while they're generally less likely to admit, also have numerous thoughts about sex throughout the day. It may be not quite that often but they still do (and while they're at it, why not think about the ways to help their guys up the ante in the bedroom).

Another thought that men find annoying is that sex for them, according to assumption, is just a way to get off. Men can easily get off. It's called *masturbation*. Most men are emotional too. Sex can be romantic and not just a physical activity with the goal of satisfying a need. This is true, by all means, but sex can also be a way to connect with other people. Not all men are barbarians or animals with nothing better to do than to just get off.

Many confess to imagining other people, celebrities mainly, while doing the deed. This is one secret that many men actually have.

The thing is, women are also guilty sometimes. This kind of thought is considered cheating by some. But as long as one does not put thoughts into actions, then there is no actual cheating or the cheating is minimal at the least.

Many guys (women, as well) also hide the truth from their current lovers about the number of sex partners they have had. In American Pie, there's this thing they call "The Rule of Three. This rule states that; the actual number of girls a guy has slept with will be whatever number he tells you divided by 3. Conversely, the number of guys a girl has slept with will be whatever she tells you time 3. But those rules aren't true all the time. People have different reasons why they don't admit their real number. Guys sometimes lessen their number to avoid being labeled a sex fiend or sometimes to shun a fight with their jealous partners. Women do so most likely to avoid being called easy. Sex is a natural thing. The number of people any person has slept with does not dictate who he or she is as a person. Some are just more open about their sexuality than others.

Part 1: The Porn Stars Method to Explosively Enlarge Your Best Friend in Only 72 Hours

Chapter 1: Introduction to Penis Enlargement

BIG is better, say many. But just as many firmly state the opposite: size doesn't matter. And then there are some who are neither here nor there, believing "it's not what you've got, but how use it that matters"

When it comes to penis size, just about everybody has got an opinion. And that's all right. Different people have different preferences.

A new study shows that women who prefer vaginal intercourse over other types of sex like it better with men with longer penises. The same feeling is echoed by women who have frequent vaginal orgasms. These women reveal they climax more easily when having sex with a man with a longer penis.

The new studies do settle the debate once and for all.

They also prove that the male anxiety about penis size is not without a good reason — bigger penis does equate to better satisfaction for many women.

This was women's perspective. What do men in general feel about penis size? (Of course, we have to ask them too — after all it is a man thing.)

Their answer is actually hardly surprising, for men being men always like it bigger.

Forty-five percent of men, a study reveals, are unhappy with the size of their penis. (Now we know what men ask for when we say to them, "Make a wish.")

So, it's all settled and proven: many women like bigger penises and many men want the same.

Now only two important questions loom large:

1. How small is small penis?

2. How do I increase my penis size?

The answers are here. Let's dig in...

How small is small penis?

When the penis is in the flaccid state, its average length, as found by several studies, is between 3.5 and 3.9 in. On the other hand, the average length of an erect penis is between 5.5 and 6.3 in, while the average girth is between 4.7 and 5.1 in.

A penis size that is smaller than the average penis length is considered small. With that said, many men with an average or slightly-better-than-average penis believe their penis is small when it isn't.

Are there specific exercises to increase penis size?

YES. Whether your penis is small or you think your penis is small, there are exercises to increase the penis size.

Numerous exercises, when done regularly and done as directed, have shown to result in an increase in the penis size substantially. However, to enjoy the benefit, the exercises must be done 5 days a week for no less than 6 months.

The changes become visible as early as 2 or 3 weeks after starting. The real gains in the size of the penis, however, are noticed after only 6 months.

You must exercise for 1 hour 5 days a week. Two days of rest is needed. (You can take a day off on two consecutive days or on two separate days.) The rest period is crucial as it is then that the cells heal and regenerate.

How does penis size increases with exercise?

Actually it's all science. And to understand how exercises increase the penis size, we must first understand the science behind penis erection.

The penis contains **corpora cavernosa,** spongy vascular chambers that run through the length of the penis, which when filled with blood leads to erection.

The penis enlargement exercises aim to expand the size of these chambers because an expansion will allow them to absorb more blood, which in turn will affect an increase in the penis size. By deliberately stretching tissues that cause erection, the exercises create a tensile strength, which, in turn, gradually causes an increase in the growth of these tissues.

Statuary Warning

While each of the exercises given is safe, you are recommended to consult your urologist before doing them, especially if you have or have had any of the following health conditions:

Diabetes

Liver Cirrhosis

Respiratory disease

Any other disease which affects the flow of blood and oxygen into the penis

Don't take these symptoms lightly:

Bubbles on the penis (happens because during exercise pressure is put on the penis for a considerable length of time)

Some soreness (may happen because of repeated pulling of the organ)

Swelling on the penis

Stop exercises immediately if one or more of the aforementioned symptoms are experienced and immediately consult an urologist. Do not resume exercises until the symptoms have disappeared completely.

Four Things You Must Do Before Performing Penis Enlargement Exercises

1. Shave off the pubic hair. We don't want you to accidentally pull it during the exercise, because it will painful.

2. Eat healthy and drink lots of water, just like you would do if you were working on your biceps.

3. Apply a moisturizer on your penis before starting. We don't recommend soap or shampoo. They can irritate the penis skin and cause redness.

4. Measure the penis. You must measure the length and circumference of penis during an erection as well as the length of penis when it's flaccid.

Chapter 2: Hormones necessary for Penis Enlargement

Human growth hormone (HGH) is produced in the pituitary gland. As you age, the pituitary gland gradually starts to generate less of the HGH, resulting in a reduction in muscle mass and bone compactness, and escalates in fat mass. However, growth hormone can be naturally increased through weight training, aerobic exercise, appropriate nutrition and rest. Weight training assists to increase the pituitary gland to liberate the growth hormone to stimulate muscle growth and hypertrophy, as well as promotes the body to use fat as energy. When muscles contract and relax during numerous sets of weight training, the body generates hefty levels of HGH to repair and restore the tissues that have been placed under strain. HGH also increases during aerobic exercise and performing at least 30 minutes of aerobic exercise five days a week at moderate to high intensity will activate the release of HGH. Though an amplified intensity stage will promote the release of the hormone, however overtraining will do the opposite and cause it not to release. For muscle growth to happen, amino acids must be accessible in the body. Amino acids located in protein assist to restore and form muscle tissue. Guzzling a well-balanced diet involving of at least 30 percent of your overall daily calories in protein is sufficient to effectively stimulate muscle growth. Protein can originate from either plant or animal sources. However, when selecting animal sources, it is best to eat lean meats such as, lean chicken breast, beef, eggs, or low-fat dairy products. Also insufficiency of sleep or overtraining will have the opposite effect on the human growth hormone. When the body does not obtain adequate sleep or is over trained, the adrenal gland discharges the stress hormone cortisol, which triggers your body to stock more fat. For your body to generate the growth hormone, sufficient sleep is essential to promote muscle growth as a result of weight training, and the target hours of sleep should be between 7-9 hours. Exercise is one of the most efficient ways to counteract many lifestyle-related diseases. Remarkably, it can also enhance your testosterone levels. New studies in obese men propose that getting involved in more physical activity was even more useful than a weight loss diet for escalating testosterone levels. Weight lifting is the greatest form of exercise to enhance testosterone and high intensity interval training (HIIT) can also be very beneficial, although all forms of exercise should work to some degree. The human body is created in such a way that it increases stem cell quantities when we participate in more physical activity.

Chapter 3: Natural techniques to enlarge your penis in 72 hours

There are several ways by which you can increase the length and girth of your penis naturally, it all depends on how well you penis can handle such enlargement methods without you having any side effects through mishandling of such natural methods. Learn which methods of natural penis enlargement you are most comfortable with.

Natural penis enlargement involves the use of natural formulations such as herbs, exercises, and devices. With the use of enlargement exercises, pumps, traction devices and extenders you can increase the size of your cock.

Mechanical Penis Enlargement-Pumps, Extenders, Weights

Mechanical penis enlargement pumps, extenders and weights are some forms of physical devices which can be used in such a way that a permanent enlargement is achieved without any form of deformation or negative side effects as long as you use them correctly. Enlargement pumps, extenders and weights will improve your erection hardness, help prevent premature ejaculation, increase the length and girth of your penis, and can help straighten a curved penis.

Penis enlargement pumps, extenders and weights are generally classified as penis traction devices. They are generally less invasive compared to other forms of penis enlargement. You can achieve an elongation of your penis by up to 25% or even more depending on the effectiveness of the traction devices. Pumps, extenders and weights are also one of the best options in the increase of penis shaft for a small penis.

The **penis enlargement pump** is a cylinder which can fit perfectly well on the length of your penis, and with the help of a manual or motorized pump, a suction effect will be created on your penis. A hand pump is more reliable because you have more control over the suction. A partial vacuum is created on your penis with these pumps, and when such vacuum is created, blood will rush through the nerves, and with continuous increase in blood pressure, you penis becomes enlarged in length and girth.

Penis extenders are also referred to as penis stretchers. These stretches will exert continuous traction on your penis. Your penis becomes can grow in length and girth. Penis extenders will extend or stretch your penis according to the period of time the device is worn (the more you wear it, the longer and wider your penis can grow). The advantage of a penis extender is that is can be worn during day under your clothes. "Hey buddy is that a pencil in your pocket or are you just happy to see me?" Just don't get caught! A penis extender contains plastic rings and metallic rods, the rods provide the traction and with an extender you can achieve an extra 2.3cm on the length of your penis but you will have to wear it for 3-4 hours every day for up to 5 months for better results. So yes it will take some time to see some gains.

Weight hanging for penis enlargement usually involves the use of attaching device which grips on the glans of the penis, the weight will be suspended over a certain period of time on your penis and the motive behind the use of weight is to increase the weight on your penis. Be sure to be cautious using this method as you should only gently increase the weight you are comfortable with as to not tear any ligaments. You can achieve extensive penis growth by hanging penis enlargement weights for several weeks at 10-20 minutes per exercise.

Supplements for Penis Enlargement

Penis enlargement pills, patches and drugs are often recommended for individuals who do not have much time for penis enlargement exercises or some other natural means of penis enlargements. Pills are quick an easy fix, which are better for sexual stamina not permanent enlargement of your penis. Size gains are only temporary. So you if you want lasting penis enlargement gains, yes you will have to take some time and dedication with exercises and using enlargement devices regularly to see significant improvement.

However keep dedicated to your penis regiment and you will see results!

The most recent and widely used penis supplement and pills comprises of two major amino acids- **L-Ornithine and L-Arginine**. These two amino acids are more common in supplements used by body builders to increase their bodies' endurances during physical activities and also speed up their recovery time. L-Argine is an amino acid produced naturally in the body, it is used in the making of penis enlargement pills because it plays a very vital role in the body's tissue and cardio-vascular health. L-arginine has been found to be capable of increasing the dilation of the blood vessels, ensuring that there is more inflow of blood in and out of the penis.

Another way through which an L-arginine supplement or pills can work for you is the substance that has been found to be capable of increasing the levels of Human Growth Hormone (HGH) in the body- this hormones help reduce stress by reducing fatigue, it is really helpful for you if your sexual dysfunction results from stress, fatigue and anxiety.

The usage of penis enlargement pills and supplements will depend on a number of factors, these include; health history of the user, the sexual life and pattern, age, and several others. A physician will ideally asked and investigate your medical history before recommending a particular penis enlargement pill or supplement for you, this will help you avoid some common problems and complications.

There are countless number of penis enlargement pills around, many of the low quality pills don't do much, you should not rely on online reviews only, contacting individuals who have actually used such pills in recent times may be your best possible way of detecting the authenticity of such products. "Hey buddy how are those penis pills working out for ya?"

Medical/surgical penis enlargement

The most common medical procedure you can use to enlarge your penis size is Phalloplasty. This surgical procedure cannot be classified as a natural penis enlargement method because it is invasive in nature. I would highly recommend against going the surgical route. Aside the fact that surgical penis enlargement may cost you a lot of money, the invasive nature of such procedures can lead to a permanent damage to the tissues of your penis. In most cases surgical penis enlargement becomes painful and may require that an individual use analgesics.

Basically, the procedure of enlarging the penis through surgical means involve the surgeon cutting out the ligaments which hold the penis in position, and then your penis will be allowed to descend. With the use of a permanent surgical extender, your penis will be permanently elongated over a period of weeks. Performing a surgical penis enlargement on your penis will help you achieve between 1-2 inches of extra length and up to 1 inch of girth extension. Penis enlargement through surgery can leave you scars as well. Your erection will normally point downwards after the surgery and who wants that?

Dermal implant is another surgical technique through which your penis can be enlarged. Dermal implant involves the transplant of some fat cells from other parts of the body on to the penis. The head of the penis cannot be enlarged may make the whole process rather odd. Aside the fact that your penis head may look absurd with cells transfer, the accumulation of fat cells in a particular region of your penis may make your penis lumpy. The main reason why a surgeon may not perform this kind of surgical penis enlargement on you is because of the side effects.

If you are planning to perform a surgical penis enlargement procedure you should be ready to part with several thousands of dollars – usually between $2,000 - $5000 or more in some cases. In several cases, a surgical operator will ask for your health insurance cover before a surgical penis enlargement procedure is performed on you, the cost implications as well as a higher tendency to develop post surgical problems are the most common reasons why medical handlers ask.

If you can't afford a surgical penis enlargement operation, or you believe you wouldn't be able to handle the post operation problems, then your best bet is to make use of safer and less invasive natural penis enlargement methods without the high cost and side effects, and will give you long term penis enlargement.

Problems with surgical operation for penis enlargement

The physical and psychological problems associated with surgical extension of the penis vary from mild to severe. Most surgical operations do come with complications. If you want to go for a surgical elongation of your penis, keep in mind that as many as 30% of those who go for surgical enlargement of penis do not feel completely satisfied with the result. Depending on the structure and nature of your penis growth, you should expect a minimum of 1 inch extension and most people do not achieve more than 2 inches. If you achieve less than 1 inch of penis growth through surgical operations, then there must be some underlying factors.

Post surgical operation infections and scarring may be witnessed during or after penis enlargement surgery. If you suffer from minor scars, such may heal over time but when such infection is turning to soreness or blisters, then you must consult your doctor for proper post-surgical operation treatment. Though your penis should heal in few days after the surgical operations, it may take several weeks in some cases. You may suffer from redness and itching while severe complications may include difficulty in urination, problems with erection and many others. You don't have to be scared of these complications as most of them will disappear in just a relatively short period of time.

Damages to surrounding tissues and nerves are also common. Some of the tissues surrounding the penis and those which take active part in the normal functioning of the penis may find it difficult to adjust to the new structure and size of the penis, in some cases they become damaged or malfunction.

There are several considerations that you must consider before choosing the ideal penis enlargement product and methods for yourself. You need to ensure that the safety of your penis as well as your general wellbeing is ensured. Most natural penis enlargement methods are safe to use, however getting the right concentration of usage or intensity will determine how safe you can use such methods and products.

You should consider the nature of your penis before deciding which enlargement product is ideal for you. If you suffer from erectile dysfunction, natural herbs might be the most suitable method for you, however if you are not suffering from any underlying health conditions such as erectile dysfunction, then you may go for mechanical devices. Treating underlying sexual conditions may be the first step towards choosing an ideal natural penis enlargement product for you.

Prices of natural penis enlargement products should have little effect on your choice of product, most herbal natural penis enlargement products come at cheaper prices compared to mechanical penis enlargement devices, though not all herbal products are cheaper than mechanical devices, this is one of the reasons why you should not allow prices of products to decide your choice of product. You should be careful of extremely cheap products that may be imitations of original products.

The best penis enlargement products should come with a limited warranty. This should include a full refund of money if the product does not cause a meaningful impact on your penis under a certain period of time. Some herbal product manufacturers will allow you to have a taste of what they have to offer for a limited period of time before you actually subscribe to buying the product package.

As per mechanical devices, it will be ideal for you to read product reviews online or ask individuals who have actually used such products to be able to determine which one that will work perfectly for you. The mechanical devices you choose must not be too fragile to break. Your mechanical device must not put any harm on your penis.

Penis enlargement pills and patches can be easily applied, but they must not trigger any form of allergic reaction. You should go for a natural penis supplements without additives. Generally be careful in your selection processes while choosing the ideal penis enlargement products for your needs. Be opened to advice from physicians, friends, and read as many reviews as possible.

Part 2: 5 Natural and Easy-to-Find Ingredients for Boost Your Sex Life and Improve Sex Duration

Chapter 1: Boosting Sex life

Note Insecurities Down

Whenever you feel insecure about something, just write it down on a piece of paper. When you do this, you are going to make the insecurity something that you can objectively analyze. When you write your insecurity down, read it back to yourself. Question this insecurity, ask yourself why you feel this way. Is the insecurity valid? Is it necessary? Try to find out the source of this insecurity, and ask yourself if that source is even trustworthy.

Eventually you will start to see that a lot of your insecurities are the result of bad perceptions of yourself. You are not actually as bad as you make yourself out to be. However, your perception of yourself remains negative. It is this aspect of your life that you will truly be able to change once you start writing down your insecurities and analyzing them.

Educate Yourself

There is a lot of shame that is commonly attributed to sex. What your preferences are, the way you feel about your body, a lot of these things are judged by people. You are made to feel unusual, a freak as it were. This is why it is so important to start educating yourself about sex. Learn about as many sexual preferences as possible. You will find out that a lot of your preferences are very commonplace. Even the most outlandish ones would be perfectly normal, with legitimate explanations. Unless you are a pedophile, it is highly unlikely that your sexual preferences will be so abhorrent that they would warrant disgust.

The fear of being judged plays a huge role in making men feel stressed out about sex. This stress usually results in erectile dysfunction more often than not.

Do Things That Make you Feel the Way You Want to Feel

We live in exciting times. People no longer have to conform to enforced notions of gender anymore. A man is no longer less of a man if he cries, and he is no longer expected to be burly and stoic. You are, essentially, freer than ever before to be whoever you want to be. This means that a lot of your stress in not valid. Most men feel stressed out because they do not conform to these notions of masculinity. It is a natural occurrence, since this is the first generation that is emerging after those imposed notions of masculinity have been removed.

The best way you can build sexual confidence is being the kind of man you want to be. There are women and men out there with incredibly diverse tastes and preferences. This means that no matter what kind of man you want to be, you can be sure that there will be a host of potential partners for you. Stop worrying about being the "right" kind of man. There is no such thing. By worrying so much about something so meaningless, you are going to end up suffering from erectile dysfunction if you are not suffering from it already.

Have More Sex

The only way you can get confident about sex is by having as much sex as possible. This might seem odd to you, but this really is the best way. If you are stressed out about sex, chances are your erectile dysfunction has not progressed to the point where you are completely unable to get erect. Even if you are, there are so many people in the world who would enjoy the kinkier side to sex that you can be sure that you would find someone willing to acquiesce to your requirements.

By having sex, you will realize that it really isn't that difficult. If you are young, there are plenty of opportunities to have sex. As long as you ensure that you are safe, having sex will help you develop a better body image as well. This is because having sex will instill in you the belief that you are not unattractive. After all, why would anyone have sex with someone unattractive?

Remove the Negatives from your Vocabulary

Being self deprecating is fair, and can be funny in some occasions. However, this is only up to the point where it is amusing and not an actual representation of what you think about yourself. If you are constantly self deprecating, you are going to end up believing some of the things you are saying. Remain positive about your body image, and avoid all negative spaces where people would make you feel bad about yourself.

This is especially important for you as a man who is suffering from erectile dysfunction. If you are in a space where you feel as though you are being ridiculed or made to feel low about your dysfunction, leave that space immediately. The stress that would come from the ridicule will greatly exacerbate your erectile dysfunction.

Look at Real Bodies

Watching porn and looking at male models might leave you with the impression that real men are ripped and muscular, and that they all have large penises. This is not the case at all. Real mean are fat and skinny, they are bald and hairy, and penis size ranges from four all the way to seven inches long. And each and every one of these men has sex. You can too, there is no reason why you are any less than any other man.

In order to form a better body image, try looking at as many real bodies as possible. Try going for amateur porn which would have normal men instead of studio porn where porn stars are chosen for their looks.

Admit the Importance of Body Positivity

For a lot of people, body image issues is something only women suffer from. As a man, you can suffer from them too. Acknowledge this fact. Stressing out over your body image issues is probably what caused your erectile dysfunction in the first place, so try to acknowledge the importance of accepting your body.

Turn on the switch

Variety is the spice of life, therefore to make yourself the desire of a woman; you must know how to spice things up, and how to explore various strategies to ensure that she receives maximum pleasure during sex.

On this note, we are going to discuss this chapter as a means to achieving two aims; the first aim is the tactical aim, that is a means to stay longer without ejaculation and the second is to be able to spice things up for maximum satisfaction.

When you are digging down your woman, always ensure that you are hitting the right note. How do I mean? Make sure that you are not the only one feeling the sensation, that your partner is also enjoying the rhythm. This could be easily known from her reaction during the sex. Though the reaction of a woman to the sensation of sex differs and it's dependent on the background and culture of the woman.

You can engage to have fun-filled time with your partner without untimely interruption from the flow of nature. I want to believe you do engage your woman with varieties of styles during sex, if not, you need to start doing it right away.

When you engage different styles, it makes you stay longer during sex. This is how it works; during the period of switching from one style to another, there is always a break when you either pause to assume another position or totally withdraw to be able to do different things from what you have been doing before. This serves as a means to ensure that you stay longer as the pressure is reduced on your penis during this short break.

At the same time, you also achieve the aim of making your woman enjoy sex with you the more because the pleasure a woman feels during sex is related to the angle at which she has been penetrated from. There are some positions you assume that put pressure on her G-spot, this kind of position makes her journey into the land of big-O very fast. For instance, when you enter your partner with her back on the ground and her two legs raised in the air in a missionary position, you are entering at an angle which gives you a hedge to be hitting the G-spot. This style is best practiced on the couch.

There are some styles you engage that put you at a vantage position to directly engage the clitoris. Doggy style is one of those styles that helps you to engage her clit; when you penetrate from the rear, you could use your hand to directly touch her clit intermittently during the penetration or in continuous fondling of her sensitive spot depending on her reaction to it, because the clit might get so sensitive during sex that it becomes painful when touched, you need to understand.

The degree to which your partner enjoys sex with you is determined by how creative you are in bed. To be more creative, you need to engage more styles during sex. At the same time, you need to be careful so you don't switch styles too often that it becomes absurd or make her feel uncomfortable. When you are engaging a style, wait to see her reaction towards the particular style, to be able to determine whether you should continue or switch. To know if she enjoys a particular style or not, you should have spent at least one to three minutes, then observe her response.

This is how you know the style you should continue or discontinue immediately, when you use a particular style and her moaning suddenly increase or you notice that she breathes faster at that point, that should send a signal to you that she is probably enjoying the position better. Then it is not the time to switch, you need to continue and even increase the pace if possible to be able to give her maximum satisfaction.

Meanwhile, you engage another position and her moaning suddenly decreases or even stop, or you begin to feel as if she is absent-minded during the engagement, it means she is bored by the position and not really enjoying it, then you might need to switch immediately.

Your switch must always be turned on during sex to maximize the game and make it optimum for your partner as the advantage is for the both of you. Naturally, some women enjoy a particular style better on bed, depending on their body structure. Some prefer the missionary position, to some; it is cow girl that does the job, to another it is doggy, while some prefer scissors, and others prefer 69 and so forth. There is nothing like "one size fit all" in the matter of sex position and styles, it varies from woman to woman.

Nonetheless, a survey was carried out among women of sexually active age, it was discovered that many women prefer doggy style based on their responses. It was also discovered that many women prefer to be in charge than to stay passive at the receiving end. Meaning that they want to be in control of the affairs during sex, cow girl, doggy and reverse cow girl are styles that fit such tendencies.

All these are opinion, the main job is to understand your woman and know what works best for her and how she loves to receive it.

SWITCH THE PACE

The switch is not only applied to your style, but also to your pace. It was discovered that your pace during sex also determines how much your partner will enjoy it. Oftentimes, the pace at which the penetration is done is dependent on the mood of the man or woman or even the environment. You will find out that when you are excited, your pace isn't slow like slot but fast and furious, and when you are not really in the mood, you just manage to go in and out slowly.

At some particular time, the environment tend to dictate the pace, maybe you are just stealing the show where a little noise will alert the next neighbor of what is going on, you tend to maintain a slow pace to save the situation. Unlike in a situation where you are as free as air, you just bang as fast as you can.

Reaction of women to pace also differs from woman to woman. Some prefer it slow and sexy, some want it fast and furious while others want to stay somewhere in the middle. That is why the point for you to know your woman cannot be overemphasized. Know your woman (KYW)

On a general note, I found out that majority of women prefer their mood to determine the pace during sex. Nevertheless, it was researched that fast paced sex achieves orgasm faster in women than the slow ones.

One of the merits of switching pace during sex is to help you control the time of ejaculation. For most men, fast pace means a quick ejaculation. Your pace also determines how long you will last in bed.

In order to control the duration of your sex, switch paces, alternate between fast and slow pace. You can start very slow, increase the pace as you proceed until you are really hitting it, maintain the tempo for a while, and then switch back to slow pace again as if in a cycle. By this practice, you will last longer on her than when you rush in with fast action and then rush out with cold feet.

As a matter of principle, don't always start penetrating with a fast pace, you could run out of energy; by the time she is already enjoying your fast rhythm, your body might start to feel as if it can't carry you any longer, your slow pace then will feel like a punishment to your woman. Therefore, start slowly and increase the momentum as you go. Practice it as if you are driving a car; increase the pace as you go.

Chapter 2: How to improve sex duration

Many men are worried about their sexual performances. They want to last longer, to make their partners feel good, to be praised for their abilities. And it is nothing wrong with that. All people want to feel good, to enjoy themselves, to feel free and happy. But what do you really expect of your sexual performance? Do you want to satisfy your partner? Do you want to be better than last time? What is your goal? Sexual performance is not only about yourself; therefore "measuring" it can be more difficult, because you have to take into account multiple factors.

Who establishes your sexual performance? Is it you or your partner? Or both? You should answer these questions to know what you have to do. Usually, men define sexual performance as the time of the intercourse. The longer they last, the better they think everything is. And this is partially true. But time isn't everything. You can improve your performance in many ways, depending on the needs of your partner and your own expectations.

First of all, you should try to relax.

Many men are obsessed with the idea of lasting longer. And, yes, women have to admit this is important, but is not everything. Other significant things are the attention for your partner, the physical touching, the connection between the two of you, the needs you and your partner have, the expectations you and your partner have. A good communication is the key to solving your sexual problems. If you can't talk to each other, if you don't know what your partner wants, you can't really improve your sexual performance.

Try to focus on satisfying your partner.

This includes talking to her, finding out what she wants, what she needs, what she likes and dislikes. This should be your first step. Then, you can focus on lasting longer. There is some practical general advice you can follow to improve your sexual performance, like paying attention to your diet, exercising, reducing stress. In a short while, you will start seeing the difference.

The good news is that you can always improve your sexual performance, if you really want it. There is no age limit, you only have to know yourself and your partner. Yes, it is annoying and frustrating to experience erectile dysfunction, but this doesn't mean it is the end of your intimate life. Consider it is only a stepping stone you need to overcome.

If you know what you have to do, your sexual performance will increase and both your partner and you will be pleased about it. Here are some tips to improve your sexual performance:

Try to be relaxed. Stop thinking you will not make it and stop worrying about your erections. This puts an additional stress on your shoulders and it will end up affecting your erections. So, try to be relaxed, to enjoy the moments you can spend with your partner. Don't think at anything else, just live the moment and forget about anything else. Try to educate your mind to live in the present, without wondering here and there without a reason.

Focus on cardiovascular exercise.

This improves your health and your sexual performance. You don't need to spend all day at the gym, thirty minutes a day are enough. Swimming and running are great methods to boost your libido and improve your erections. You can also practice other types of sports, depending on what you like. The most important thing is to exercise, to train your body and your mind, at the same time. This makes you feel healthy and be healthy.

Include in your diet the following: garlic, onion, bananas, chilies and peppers, omega-3 acids, eggs, vitamin B1. These contribute to your health and can significantly improve your sexual life.

Get some sun. This makes you feel better and is an excellent boost for your sexual desire. So don't stay inside, get out and enjoy your time. Fresh air is great for increasing your libido, especially summer days and nights. You can think of a vacation together with your partner in a hot destination, where you can practice every-thing you learn in this book.

Masturbation can help you last longer in bed. Before having sex with your partner, you can practice masturbation.

Connect with your partner.

A great sexual experience involves the two of you. Therefore, don't focus only on your performance, because this will make your partner feel unimportant. Focus on making her feel relaxed, on do-ing the things she likes. As long as you are not constantly thinking on how to last longer, things will become better.

See a sexologist.

This can be a very good way to learn more about yourself, your sexuality and what you can do to improve your intimate life. You can bring your partner with you and discuss about your problems and your expectations. There is nothing to feel ashamed about. Imagine, these people have to do this every day and they probably heard many things during their careers. So try to be honest and see this experience as an opportunity to find out new things and resolve your problems.

Try new things.

Routine is the enemy of a great sexual life, so do the best you can to avoid it. Try changing the place, the way you dress, try role-playing, whatever keeps you away from routine. Talk to your partner about what you should improve and do the best you can to come to an agreement. A relationship needs time and communication; is not something you can easily do or understand.

Increase your self-confidence.

Usually, women are more likely to have low self-confidence, but this can also happen to men. If you don't trust yourself, if you are thinking on how to last longer and can't get relaxed, you will only make things worse. To increase your self-confidence, try to adopt a positive attitude; do something for yourself, like buying a nice jacket or a new perfume, cut your hair in a different way. See what makes you feel good about yourself, because this will also increase your self-confidence and improve your sexual performance.

Try different positions.

In order to avoid routine and discover new ways of enjoying your intimate life, you should try new positions. Talk to your partner about her fantasies, about what she would like to try, tell her about your own fantasies and try new things. Establish a line you are not allowed to cross, according to your wishes.

Practice Kegel exercises.

They have many benefits and can be practiced by both men and women. You can do them anywhere, at home, while driving, while cooking, at your office or anywhere else. Tighten your pelvic muscle and keep the contraction for a couple of seconds before releasing. You should repeat at least 10 times for a set and you can do multiple sets every day. In time, this improves your erections and makes you able to control yourself for a longer period of time.

Be patient.

If you are going through a difficult time at work, give yourself the time to overcome the problem. Don't expect things to solve immediately and don't become a pessimistic. Instead, try to focus on finding a solution for your problem, without blaming yourself. Even if you decide to see a doctor, don't expect things to change within a week. It takes time to find out what is going wrong, what you should do and it is important to know you can count on the support of your partner.

Never give up.

Sometimes, it takes time to discover the cause of erectile dysfunction and this can be quite frustrating. You may need to try several treatments, but you should not give up. It is only a matter of time and will to succeed. Trial and error is sometimes inevitable, if you aren't lucky enough to get the perfect treatment from the very first time.

You can try supplements or special food to increase your libido, but only with the doctor's recommendation. Don't take supplements without consulting a doctor, because they can have many side effects and interfere with other medication you are taking. They can affect your heart and the well-functioning of your body. As much as you would like to believe they are the answer to your problems, this is rarely the case. Don't play games with your health. If you want to avoid this, always see a doctor before taking supplements.

Stay focused

A major bane of poor performance among men from the perspective of the women is self-centered sex. Sex could be self-centered especially from men, it is surprising how some men set examination by themselves, score the script and organize an award ceremony for themselves. This is true about guys who boast of how great they are in bed without realizing that the performance is only being endured by the partner.

Great sex is not defined from one angle alone. You can't say you are good in bed because you do enjoy the feelings. The question is; does your partner enjoy the act, or she is just trying to get along so that your ego will not be affected? Great sex is measured by how satisfied are the parties involved, did you both enjoy the ride? If you are given a chance in the next few hours, will you love to have same kind of feeling again?

This is one of the secrets of becoming the desire of a woman. The way you love to enjoy the sweet sensation of orgasm is the exact way a woman wants to enjoy it too, if not more. Most men concentrate on themselves and their attention is only on the time they will ejaculate.

If you can have a paradigm shift from this moment and ensure that every sexual encounter with your partner will be all about her, you will see how she will begin to desire the time with you.

A client shared with me on how his wife does not like to go down with him in bed. He concluded that his wife hates sex because she refuses most of his sexual advances. It became a tension in their home and the marriage was almost falling apart. When I interviewed the man about how long he desires to have sex with his wife, his response indicated that he wants sex almost every day or if possible twice a day. I further probed him about how many times at least in a week does his wife reach climax during sex, from his response, he was not sure if the wife has ever experienced orgasm in their marriage. I was not surprised by this response because many women above the age of forty are yet to experience orgasm for once according to a survey.

If you are in the class of men who engage in self-centered sexual intercourse, you need to stop it now. Such an act is counterproductive.

Sex should bring about mutual pleasure to the people involved; it should not be a one-sided thing. Many a times, the women are free from this guilt of self-centeredness in sex even though we have some women who are also self-centered in bed, but it is more pronounced among men because the point of orgasm of a man is easy to come by unlike that of woman who requires constant efforts, skills and experience.

As a man, how good you are in bed is determined by how good she feels during each encounter with you. Having realized this, you need to learn how to always make her feel good during sex with you. Please, don't put yourself under pressure as pressure itself has a way of sabotaging your effort and make it counterproductive. The key is for you to keep getting better every day until you become a 'pro'.

Can you imagine your partner getting to orgasm at every encounter? It will tell on her general outlook as we will be happier than those who hardly experience orgasm. It makes your partner look younger and it gives freshness to her skin. The glow on her face alone after sex and the big smile that follows is enough to convince you to always desire to make her climax at every encounter.

A major factor in becoming the desire of your woman is to focus the attention on her pleasure, let her enjoyment become your priority. Have sex as if you have no stake in it, let your attention be on her, be determined to always make your partner enjoy sex. As you think about sex, think of her interest first and how you can take her to the climax where she will like to be ever time.

Just as I explained in the past chapter about how sex starts from the mind of a woman, engage her mind to focus on sex for the moment. For example, during your normal discussion, you could just bring up some erotic conversation and ask of her opinion. Sex might be the least on her mind at that moment, but this will make her begin to think of sex and probably begin to prepare her mind to enjoy sex with you. Research has it that an average man thinks about sex nineteen times a day while an average woman thinks about sex ten times a day. That is why as a man, you should have a way of preparing her for sex.

Having done that, when the time comes for the real deal; take it slowly. Be gentle, polite and caring. You might be wondering why I am detailing the process; from experience, I have learnt that many men are very clumsy in bed; they rush the entire process and lose the very reason for the act. Therefore, one cannot over emphasize the point that you need to take time to enjoy the entire process each time you want to get down with your woman.

It is good to start with pillow talk, the heart to heart discussion that reveals things that are bugging her mind, it may be stress from her place of work or the children's health or whatever, the heart to heart discussion will help free her mind from the stress and worries to be able to concentrate on the pleasure of the moment. Note that if this process is skipped and she still has things bothering her, it might hinder her ability to climax. When sex is performed with an open mind, it enhances her ability to cum quickly.

After the discussion, move to foreplay and continue from there, as discussed in a previous chapter.

Great sex is a possibility, channel your energy towards giving her pleasure and she will want to be with you every moment of her life and you will also observe that she's becoming more protective of you, she won't want any other woman share from the kind of pleasure she is receiving. That's the beauty of becoming an action man.

Chapter 3: Ingredients to boost sex life and duration

Since a big chunk of erectile dysfunction is physiological, it stands to follow that good nutrition is key to addressing the issue. Great nutrition is all about wise eating habits and choices. Unfortunately, it isn't always possible to get all the necessary nutrients by simply eating the right foods. Often times, supplementation is needed. Eating right for addressing or reducing the risks for erectile dysfunction may require taking supplements for optimal penile health. Truth is, natural supplements, e.g., herbs, have been used since time immemorial in addressing erectile issues by African and Chinese cultures.

Compared to prescription medications for treating erectile dysfunctions such as Cialis (tadalafil), Levitra (vardenafil) and Viagra (sildenafil), supplements don't have as extensive studies or tests to back up their efficacy claims. As the amount and type of active ingredients among different erectile dysfunction supplements may vary, their side effects do so as well.

Because supplementation can be quite helpful to address erectile dysfunctions, here's a guide for choosing erectile dysfunction supplements:

Generally safe, with positive results from studies of people

➤   DHEA: There's some amount of evidence showing its ability to address erectile dysfunction. Generally safe at low doses but have been reported to cause acne in some cases.

➤   L-ARGININE: There's some evidence establishing its ability to stimulate wider blood vessel opening to increase blood flow. In some cases, it's been reported to cause diarrhea, cramps and nausea. Avoid taking together with Viagra.

➤   GINSENG: Panax ginseng has been shown in one study to improve sexual function for men who suffer from erectile dysfunction. It's cream form – applied topically – can help prevent premature ejaculation. Although generally safe for short-term use, using panax ginseng as a supplement can cause insomnia for some people.

With positive results from studies of people but higher risk

➤   YOHIMBE: Some clinical studies have shown yohimbe to help improve erectile dysfunctions brought about by antidepressant medications but have also been reported to cause relatively serious side effects in some people like anxiety, irregular heartbeat and elevated blood pressure. As such, this supplement should only be taken with approval from a licensed physician.

No significant studies on people

➤   GINGKO: This herbal supplement has good potential to improve penile blood flow but no solid evidence exists regarding claims of effectively addressing erectile dysfunction. A potential side effect of this herbal supplement is risk for bleeding.

➤   HORNY GOAT WEED (EPIMEDIUM): Although the leaves of this herb contain ingredients that are used for better sexual performance, there are no established studies on people that support the belief in its efficacy. A bonus side effect of this herbal supplement is it can help lower blood pressure.

Other non-prescription herbal alternatives

Several herbal products that claim to be the "natural" Viagra proliferate the market. The thing is, these products have undisclosed quantities of potent ingredients that are also found in their supposed synthetic counterparts and thus have higher risks for unwanted side effects. In fact, some of these products actually contain the very drugs that their supposed synthetic counterparts have that require a doctor's prescription to consume! In this case, it's best to be very vigilant in taking "herbal" erectile dysfunction supplements from manufacturers that aren't well known or don't have a good reputation in the market. Even if the FDA has banned such "herbal" supplements, they continue to proliferate illegally.

Remember, it's not enough that manufacturers claim that theirs are herbal – it's easy to claim such stuff without backing them up. Because it's practically impossible for ordinary consumers like you and I to distinguish, it's best to stick with relatively more expensive brands of herbal supplements from well-established manufacturers.

Being labeled "herbal" doesn't necessarily mean safe. Remember, they may be say taken as is but some of them may react negatively if taken with other medications. As such, it's best to consult with a licensed physician first prior to taking such supplements for erectile dysfunction, especially when taking regular medications.

Online purchase risks

With the proliferation of many online stores these days and the convenience shopping on such stores brings, no wonder many people choose to buy their supplements online. Beware though – many supplements for erectile dysfunction that are sold online these days contain ingredients that need prescription or worse, are undisclosed.

Many men who purchase erectile dysfunction supplements online think these are safe because of the nice packaging. These are often labeled as "all-natural" or "safer than prescription medicines but are just as effective." The scary truth is often times, the label tells a different story than the content. The worse thing that can happen is that these supplements contain dangerous ingredients that aren't on the label. In fact, the United States Food And Drugs Administration (FDA) – through its Internet and Health Fraud division – conducted an online survey that revealed more than 1/3 of erectile dysfunction supplements purchased online contained prescription grade ingredients and other similar substances that weren't even disclosed.

Two of these are the ingredients sildenafil and vardenafil (or substances very similar to these), the active ingredients for Viagra and Levitra, respectively. If people who have issues with Viagra and Levitra take these supplements thinking they're safer than the two prescription medicines, they may be in for a rude awakening as they suffer from side effects that they're trying to avoid in the first place.

What's more, even if the men taking these supplements have no issues with Viagra or Levitra, it's possible for them to suffer adverse side effects if they're taking medicines that don't mix well with the 2 prescription medicines' active ingredients that aren't disclosed in the supplements. For example, if a person is taking prescription medicine that contains nitrates, taking supplements that unknowingly contain sildenafil (an active component of Viagra) may bring down his blood pressure dangerously low. Nitrates are a common ingredient in prescription medicines used to treat or manage heart disease, high cholesterol, high blood pressure and diabetes and incidentally, men who are being treated for these conditions also suffer from erectile dysfunction.

Non-oral solutions for erectile dysfunction

Until recently, medical or supplemental treatments for erectile dysfunction were taken orally. Although those may work well for many, there are some men who aren't predisposed to the ingredients of such medicines or supplements, especially those who take prescription medicines that contain nitrates. Oral treatments may also have side effects that can negate the erection benefits offered.

Now, non-oral treatments are available for erectile dysfunctions as an alternative to oral treatments. They vary in efficacy and side effects. To help you sift through them, here's a list of the most popular topical solutions for erectile dysfunction:

➤ AndroGel: Many cases of erectile dysfunctions are caused by low testosterone levels. One of the most popular ways of addressing this deficiency is testosterone replacement but technically, it doesn't help men with normal levels of testosterone and those who suffer from erectile dysfunction. Testosterone can also be delivered by skin application via AndroGel – testosterone in a gel. Some of the potential side effects worth noting are emotional instability, acne and headache.

➤ Alprostadil: This kind of topical solution is classified as a vasodilator, substances that can help blood vessels to expand and improve blood flow. Since erectile dysfunction is physically a blood flow issue, Alprostadil is used for treating erectile dysfunction and is administered directly via injection into the penis or suppository insertion into the urethra. In has a reported efficacy rate of about 80%. There are no known side effects.

Alprostadil is also available as a topically applied solution, which spares men from penile scarring, bleeding and bruising. Tests have confirmed that it helps in most erectile dysfunction cases with minimal and tolerable side effects.

Chapter 4: Nutririon for Penis Enlargement

Supplements can be ingested in numerous structures, either through pills or supplements, entire sustenances, teas, herbs, and so forth... It is essential to illuminate that supplements alone will never for all time enlarge your penis. Be that as it may, appropriate supplementation can extraordinarily AFFECT THE RATE OF PENIS GROWTH while executing a penis enlargement schedule.

These 8 components are the basic variables in amplifying the impacts of a penis enlargement schedule. They can each be actuated through different means utilizing a portion of the supplements we have recorded underneath.

The response to this is troublesome, and the reason is straightforward. For the sake of science, we can not ensure that a supplement will give the fancied impacts, unless it is clinically demonstrated. The procedure of clinically demonstrating something to work, particularly in the realm of nourishment, is extremely troublesome for some reasons. All things considered, on the grounds that something has no 'logical approval', does not imply that it is not successful.

Many supplements are guaranteed to have the wanted impacts that improve penis enlargement. Luckily some of them really have investigative backing, yet numerous don't. On this site we break down whatever number of these supplements as could be expected under the circumstances and give you our legitimate knowledge on every one. The following is a rundown of all supplements that have been found in several penis enlargement or male upgrade supplements.

Eating appropriately has numerous huge medical advantages, including noteworthy penis enlargement advantages. The accompanying penis enlargement sustenances can offer you some assistance with getting the additional bigness and length size you have been longing for. Also, not at all like over-the-counter penis enlargement tranquilizes, these penis enlargement nourishments are sheltered, shabby, and sound.

You will know more need to stress over unsafe substances, unnerving symptoms, and paying a fortune. Furthermore, if that wasn't already enough, we tossed in our suggested penis enlargement vitamins too! Do you know of any penis enlargement nourishments that we disregarded? Tell us in the remark area beneath!

Lifestyle For Your Penis

Writing about a healthy lifestyle alone can fill several books. Therefore, I can only give a brief overview of how your lifestyle affects the erection or the size of your penis. But you will have realized it by now and it's hardly surprising: the way you live, will have an impact on your penis! Just in case you are already feeling resistance when reading these lines, because you do not want to give up cherished practices, that is of course fine. Nonetheless, remind yourself quickly, what pleasures you can gain through all of that! Even if a higher life expectancy alone is not a cause for change, maybe you will be convinced by great sex and larger sex stamina until old age?

1. **Smoking**:

Smoking is not only harmful to your overall health, but endangers your penis as well - at least its growth in size and its ability to have erections. **Because smoking decreases the blood flow**! This is also the very reason why smokers often have cold hands. And you do know what happens when there is low blood flow in your penis, right?!

2. **Stress**:

Stress is the cause of many diseases and the No. 1 cause of death in the United States. Therefore, it makes sense to reduce or avoid stress in your life wherever it is possible. Similarly, if you have ever tried to have sex when you were under tremendous stress, then you know what I mean. You may want it a lot, and stand across from the most beautiful woman, but still your body is not cooperating. The result: Your penis is limp. Embarrassing as this is, it is also, unnecessary. Because stress is avoidable, becaus we allow us to be stressed through other people, bad time management, wrong priorities, etc. But for the benefits of your cock, start making different decisions to improve things on a basic level.

3. **Sleep**:

Let me say this clearly: too little sleep can be absolutely devastating for your sex life! If you are so tired that you cannot think straight, your penis is guaranteed to not be in top form. If you can barely stand up straight from sheer weariness, how should your cock do it successfully then? And let's just assume that it somehow pulls itself together - just for you – obviously there will be no peak performance. So, if you prefer your erections to be rock hard and to remain like that, ensure adequate sleep.

4. **Mindset**:

Do you want a long, thick, rock hard cock permanently? I'll tell you how to get it...

It's simple: you have to believe that it works! Stop with all the self-doubt. Stop the inner critic who bullies you at every opportunity (and laughs at your penis). Once you believe in your success, take concrete actions and stick to it until you have reached your goal, then you will inevitably have success.

And there is an extra bonus on top of it all: Did you know that you will automatically increase your self-confidence by doing so? And this special boost in confidence it not due to the increased size of your cock.

Because the more consistent you are doing something with self-discipline, the more confident you become. You can start relying on yourself. And isn't this great?

5. **Fitness**:

The proper strength training makes you manly and releases testosterone. You can support the penis exercise with it, provided it is intense enough to stimulate the natural production of testosterone and muscle growth. Pick an exercise program where you are working with heavier weights and small number of repetitions. Very deliberate and slow exercises are particularly effective at promoting testosterone production, because they provide good muscle build up.

6. **Diet**:

If you want faster or better results, this is THE alternative for you! Eat the right foods and spice up your diet with additional matching supplements of purely natural origin and your progress will accelerate tremendously. In so doing significantly more growth is possible - in a safe and healthy manner. This way the blood will be enriched with all the improved nutrient supply, which promotes rapid growth.

If you do now the exercises described here, the chemically enriched blood will flow increasingly into the penis, and all those substances will be made available and encourage your penis to grow and become larger. The longer you can keep up the erection then, the more you will benefit from the high-quality nutrients, with which the blood is enriched.

Measure, But Do it Correctly

Do not overdo it!

Let me repeat it here again: Please, do not overdo it with the exercises. Impatience gives you nothing but harm! Stay persistent and do the exercises regularly. Then you will succeed and see significant progress.

Do you really want to up the ante and accelerate your penis growth and give it more inches? Then there is only one way to do it that is effective and safe: Change your diet! Because, as already mentioned, an increased supply of nutrients accelerates the growth process. And that is the only sensible, safe and healthy way to speed things up.

Regular Measurements

a. **Do not measure daily**: Of course you are interested in how much progress is achieved, and if your dick has finally become longer, but still, do not measure it every day! Because, even if you gain, for example, 8 mm in 2 months, this corresponds to a growth of only 0.13 mm per day. It is impossible to measure these small daily increases.

b. **Exactly defined intervals**: Select a specific time interval, for example, every 3-4 weeks where you regularly measure. Would you like to do it even better? Take on that day 3 different measurements and calculate the average. In this way, you compensate for fluctuations, because no man has always the same erection!

c. **Always measure in the same way**: This is actually the most important thing, because then you minimize measurement errors.

Always measure in the same position (sitting, standing or lying down)

Always use the same ruler (no set square, or a ruler that rolls up)

Make sure to always get the same angle of the penis to the ground

Last but not least: Learn to measure correctly!

Various measurement methods

BPEL - Bone Pressed Erect Length: This method is relatively accurate, and is, therefore, most frequently used. Once you have reached full erection, take the ruler and press it over the base of the penis directly against the abdomen on to the pelvic bone. Therefore the name "Bone Pressed".

NBPEL - None Bone Pressed Erect Length: Only the visible, erect penis length is measured, which begins outside the skin. Unlike BPEL, do not force the ruler against the pelvic bone, but put it down only slightly on the abdomen. **(This method is more inaccurate.)**

BPFL - Bone Pressed Flaccid Length: Here the penis is measured in the soft state. As with the BPEL also, place the ruler at the base of the penis and press it against the pelvic bone. However, it is often difficult to measure the penis size when flaccid, because many factors can affect the penis! Think only of the cold water in the swimming pool. **(This method is also more inaccurate.)**

BPFSL - Bone Pressed Flaccid Stretched Length: The penis is flaccid. You put the ruler right next to the base of the penis, and press it against the abdomen or pelvic bone. Then, pull on the penis until it reaches its maximum length. In this way, you "simulate" the erect length of the penis. Usually, the thus measured length corresponds surprisingly accurately to the actual erect penis length. It is a relatively safe indication that the penis enlargement exercises work, if this measuring method shows a change. In this way, progress can most immediately be recognized, even if the actual growth in the erect penis can often only be seen a little later.

EG - Erect Girth: This way, you measure the girth of your penis. For that, you just put a tape measure around the erect penis and measure either at the base of the penis, in the middle or just below the glans! Always measure at the same place.

Penis diameter: If you want the exact diameter of your penis, use the following formula: diameter = circumference / Pi (Pi is 3.1415). If you now have a penis circumference of 10 cm, the diameter of your penis: 3.18 cm (10 cm /3.1415)

Conclusion

Wherever you are standing at this moment, you are holding in your hands, a working system, with which you too can train your penis up to your desired size. The techniques presented herein are proven to work and have helped thousands of men grow their penis by several inches - in extreme cases to even grow up to 4 inches.

But there is a price to pay: you have to work for it and you need patience with yourself. Because, the growth phase of every man is different! So don't look for immediate results, go for the long term gain. You CAN do it too!

Also is a harder training not necessarily better, but can be dangerous. You are responsible for your health. These exercises are very safe, if they are properly applied. Stop immediately, if you feel any discomfort or perhaps even pain during an exercise, and increase the intensity slowly!

In addition to the aforementioned techniques, you have learned other factors that influence the growth of your penis. And if you take all the teachings and exercises seriously and keep at it, the reward is not only an impressive penis, but a rock hard erection and a better sex! In front of you lies a truly happy sex life, with a penis of which, up to now, you have only dreamt of!

All the best!

CPSIA information can be obtained
at www.ICGtesting.com
Printed in the USA
BVHW092334290421
606133BV00009B/1188

9 781801 846370